ALKALINE SMOOTHIE RECIPE

Simple and Delicious Recipes for Optimal Health and pH Balance.

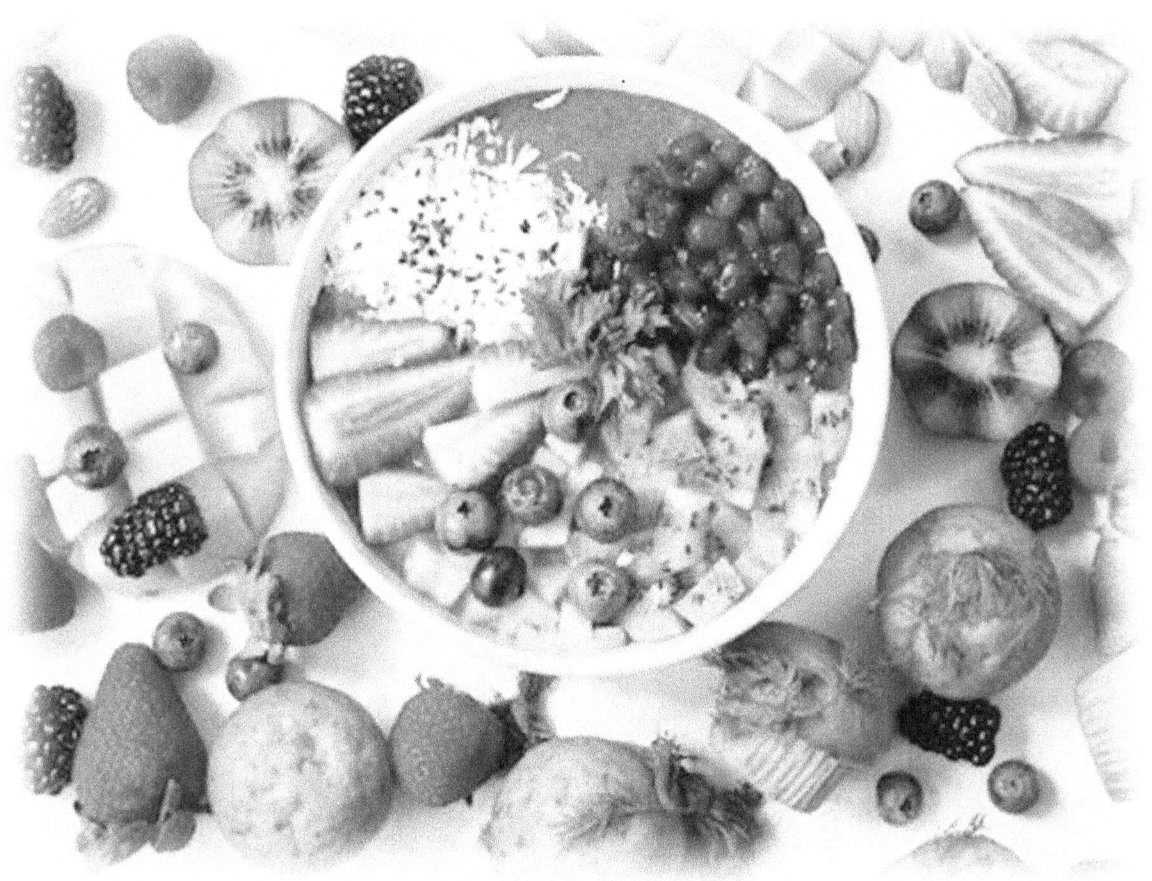

Christiana White

GAIN ACCESS TO MORE BOOKS

DISCLAIMER

The recipes in this cookbook are provided for informational purposes only and are not intended as medical or professional advice. While the author and publisher have made every effort to ensure the accuracy and effectiveness of the recipes, they are not responsible for any adverse effects r consequences resulting from the use of the suggestions herein.

The information in this cookbook should not replace professional advice. Readers are advised to consult a healthcare provider or a culinary professional before making any significant changes to their diet or cooking practices.

Nutritional information is approximate and should be used as a guide only. Variations may occur due to product availability, food preparation, portion size, and other factors.

The author and publisher disclaim any liability in connection with the use of this information. It is the reader's responsibility to determine the value and quality of any recipe or instructions provided for food preparation and to determine the nutritional adequacy of the food to be consumed.

ABOUT THE AUTHOR

When it comes to tasty and nutritious cookbooks that turn wellness into a delightful journey, Christiana White is the author you turn to. She approaches cooking from a new angle and has a passion for creating wholesome food.

Motivated by her own pursuit of health, Christiana's books on Amazon are brimming with delectable recipes that demonstrate that eating healthily can be both simple and enjoyable. Her creative method makes cooking approachable to all skill levels by fusing entire, simple foods with flavors from around the world.

Readers of Christiana's meals gush about the beneficial effects her foods have on their lives outside of the kitchen. Her books are more than just recipes; they're guides for a happier, better way of life, resulting in everything from more energy to a revitalized passion for cooking.

Come along with Christiana to discover how to turn your meals into satisfying and joyful experiences. Discover the delightful intersection of health and flavor by delving into the colourful world of her cookbooks.

TABLE OF CONTENTS.

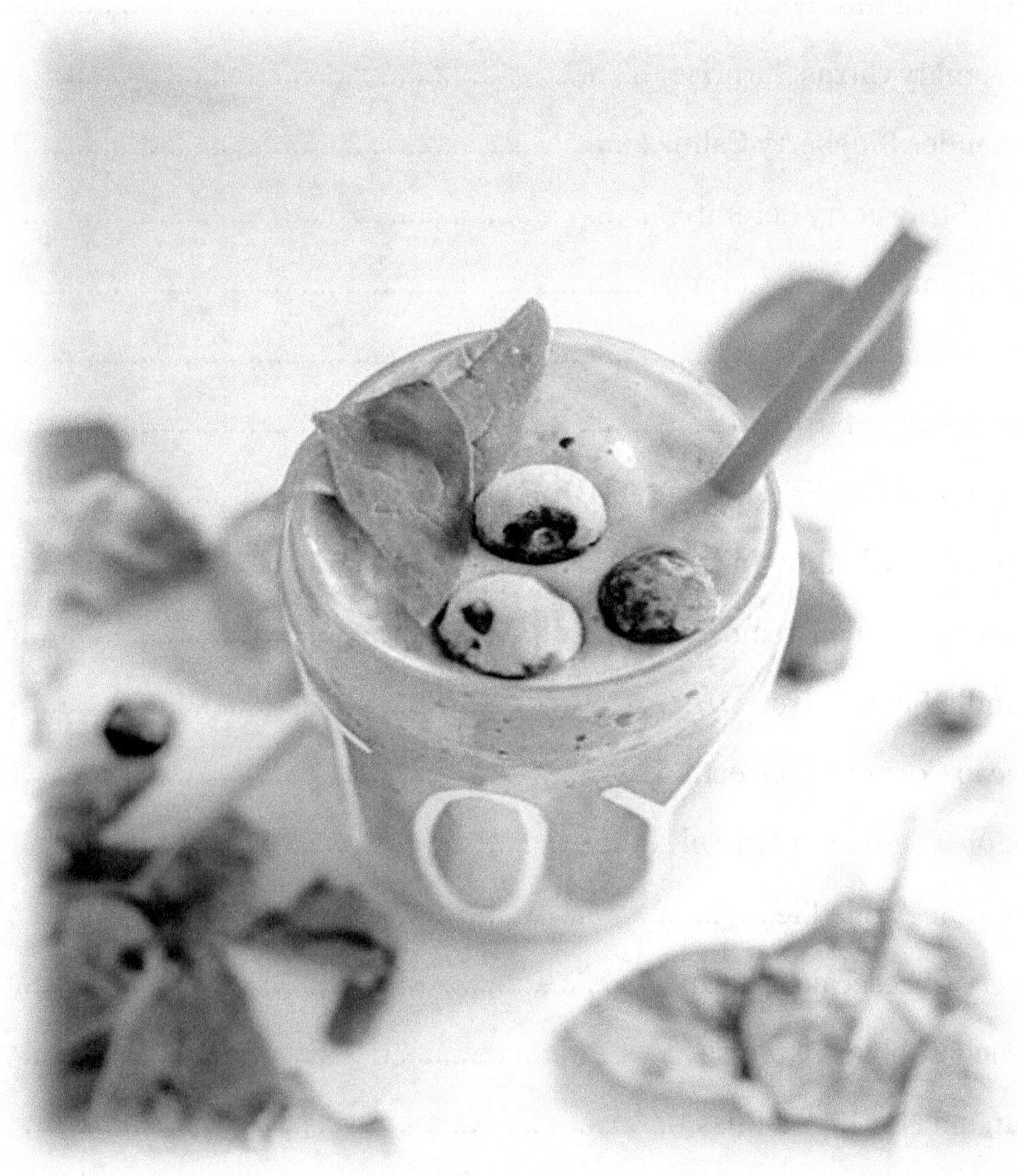

INTRODUCTION

Are you prepared to reach your body's maximum potential? Imagine waking up every morning feeling refreshed, energized, and ready to face the world. Imagine yourself effortlessly maintaining a healthy weight, gorgeous skin, and a digestive system that operates flawlessly. Doesn't that sound incredible?

Well, I'm here to tell you that it's not simply a dream. This is the power of the alkaline smoothie lifestyle.

These vivid cocktails, backed by research and powered by the extraordinary nutrient density of fruits, vegetables, and other alkalizing components, have the potential to alter your health from inside. Alkaline smoothies can boost your energy levels, improve your digestion, and even help you lose weight by neutralizing excess acid, lowering inflammation, and infusing your body with vital nutrients.

However, this is more than just looking and feeling well; it is about fostering a deep sense of well-being that radiates from inside. The alkaline smoothie lifestyle is more than simply a diet; it's a journey to a more vibrant, healthier you.

Are you ready to start on a journey that will transform the way you think about food and provide your body with the sustenance it requires? The recipes and advice in this book will guide you to a brighter, more invigorated future. It's time to take the first step towards reaching your full potential and living a healthy life.

<u>**The Power of Alkaline Smoothies**</u>

Alkaline smoothies are more than just a trendy health craze; they're a delicious and effective way to improve your health from the inside out. These vivid blends take advantage of the inherent alkalinity of fruits, vegetables, and other nutrient-dense ingredients to produce a symphony of flavor and health benefits that can transform your daily routine.

So, what makes alkaline smoothies special?

- pH Balancing: The modern diet, which is often high in processed foods, sugar, and unhealthy fats, can result in an overly acidic environment in the body. This acidity has been related to a wide range of health problems, including inflammation, exhaustion, and decreased immunity. Alkaline smoothies help to balance out the acidity by delivering alkalizing minerals and nutrients that support good health.
- Nutrient Powerhouses: Alkaline smoothies are high in vitamins, minerals, antioxidants, and fiber, providing a concentrated dose of nutrients with each sip. From leafy greens like kale and spinach to vivid berries and tropical fruits, each item has its own nutritional profile and works synergistically to support your body's important activities.
- Energy Boost: Unlike sugary drinks and processed snacks, which cause a sugar rush followed by a crash, alkaline smoothies deliver lasting energy. This is due to the complex carbohydrates found in fruits and vegetables, which the body slowly breaks down, releasing energy throughout the day.

- Detoxification Support: Many alkaline substances, such as lemon, ginger, and cucumber, are naturally detoxifying. These compounds can aid in your body's natural detoxification processes, removing toxins and promoting a cleaner interior environment.
- Weight Management: By substituting sugary drinks and harmful snacks with alkaline smoothies, you are not only providing your body with important nutrients, but also lowering your overall calorie consumption. The fiber in these smoothies promotes satiety, keeping you fuller for longer and decreasing cravings.

Beyond the obvious health benefits, alkaline smoothies are enjoyable to make and consume. Experimenting with diverse combinations of fruits, vegetables, herbs, and spices allows you to create distinct flavor profiles that both tickle your taste buds and nourish your spirit. Whether you want a brilliant green smoothie with leafy greens or a tropical fruit blend filled with sunshine, there is an alkaline smoothie recipe for everyone.

In essence, alkaline smoothies are a tasty and easy approach to adopt a healthy lifestyle. Incorporating them into your daily routine is more than just drinking a smoothie; it is an investment in your long-term health and well-being. Let the brilliant colors, refreshing Flavors, and potent nutrients of alkaline smoothies revive and awaken your senses.

CHAPTER 1: ALKALINE DIET ESSENTIALS

What is the Alkaline Diet?

The alkaline diet, also known as the acid-alkaline or alkaline ash diet, is a dietary plan that emphasizes eating items that are thought to have an alkalizing effect on the body. The theory of this diet is that the foods we eat can affect the pH balance of our physiological fluids, such as blood and urine.

The pH scale goes from 0 to 14, where 0 is the most acidic, 7 is neutral, and 14 is the most alkaline. Proponents of the alkaline diet think that a slightly alkaline internal environment (blood pH of 7.35-7.45) is best for health and wellness.

How does this diet work?

The alkaline diet classifies foods based on their ability to produce acidic or alkaline byproducts (ash) during digestion and metabolism. Meat, poultry, fish, dairy, eggs, grains, and processed meals are acidic, whereas fruits, vegetables, nuts, seeds, and some legumes are alkaline

To maintain a slightly alkaline condition in the body, the diet recommends eating more alkaline-forming foods (around 80%) and fewer acid-forming foods (20%).

What are the limitations and criticisms?

- While some research reveals possible benefits, the scientific evidence for the alkaline diet's effectiveness remains limited and unclear.
- Oversimplification of pH balance: The body's pH is closely maintained by a variety of systems, and diet has little impact on blood pH.
- Restrictive nature: The diet removes or restricts particular food groups, making it difficult to maintain long-term and perhaps leading to nutrient shortages.
- Misinformation: Some proponents of the alkaline diet make exaggerated claims about its benefits, which can lead to confusion.

Should you try it?

If you're thinking about trying the alkaline diet, talk to a doctor or a qualified dietician first. They can assist you in determining its suitability for your specific needs and goals, as well as guiding you through making informed food choices to guarantee a balanced and nutritious diet.

It's vital to note that the alkaline diet is not a cure-all for health. A balanced, whole-foods diet high in fruits, vegetables, and other nutrient-dense meals is typically suggested for overall health and well-being, regardless of how it affects pH levels.

Benefits of Alkaline Smoothies

Incorporating alkaline smoothies into your daily routine can help you achieve maximum health and well-being. These bright mixtures provide numerous benefits in addition to their delightful flavor. Let's look at the many benefits of drinking these alkalizing elixirs:

1. Restored pH Balance: A modern diet high in processed foods, sweets, and bad fats can alter your body's sensitive pH balance, resulting in an overly acidic environment. This acidity has been related to a number of health concerns, including inflammation, exhaustion, and weakened immunity. Alkaline smoothies balance out the acidity by delivering alkalizing minerals and nutrients that promote a better internal environment.

2. Increased Energy: Forget the sugar-induced energy collapses that come with sugary drinks and processed foods. Alkaline smoothies provide prolonged energy that keeps your body going throughout the day. This is due to the complex carbohydrates found in fruits and vegetables, which are slowly broken down by the body and release energy over time. Furthermore, the high concentration of vitamins and minerals in these smoothies nourishes your cells and promotes proper cellular function, increasing your energy levels.

3. Improved Digestion: The fiber component of alkaline smoothies contributes significantly to digestive health. Fiber increases stool bulk, allowing for smoother bowel movements and reducing constipation. It also functions as a prebiotic, nourishing beneficial bacteria in your gut and supporting a healthy gut microbiota, both of which are necessary for proper digestion and nutrient absorption.

4. Reduced Inflammation: Chronic inflammation is a silent cause of many health issues, including heart disease, arthritis, and autoimmune illnesses. Alkaline smoothies contain anti-inflammatory chemicals found in fruits, vegetables, and herbs. These substances assist to neutralize free radicals, reduce oxidative stress, and reduce inflammation, potentially lowering the risk of chronic disease and improving general health.

5. Weight Management: Are you struggling to maintain a healthy weight? Alkaline smoothies can be an effective weight-management aid. They are naturally low in calories and high in fiber, so you'll feel satisfied for longer and have fewer cravings. By substituting sugary drinks and bad snacks with nutrient-dense smoothies, you can fuel your body while keeping your calorie count under control.

6. Glowing Skin: The adage "you are what you eat" is especially relevant when it comes to your skin. Alkaline smoothies have a wealth of vitamins, minerals, and antioxidants that nourish your skin from within, creating a healthy glow and decreasing the signs of aging. These nutrients protect your skin from free radicals, pollution, and UV radiation, resulting in a glowing complexion.

7. Boosted Immunity: The vitamins, minerals, and antioxidants in alkaline smoothies work together to strengthen your immune system. They promote the formation of immune cells, improve their function, and protect them from harm, making you more resistant to infections and illnesses. Consuming these nutrient-rich mixtures on a regular basis provides your immune system with the tools it requires to successfully defend your body.

8. Improved Mood and Mental Clarity: Because of its complex relationship with your mental and emotional well-being, a healthy gut is frequently referred to as the "second brain." Alkaline smoothies, with their high fiber content and gut-friendly ingredients, promote a healthy gut microbiota, which can boost your mood, reduce anxiety, and increase mental clarity.

Alkaline smoothies provide a holistic approach to health by treating multiple aspects of your well-being at once. By including these vivid mixes into your daily routine, you are not only fueling your body, but also investing in a healthier, happier, and more vibrant lifestyle.

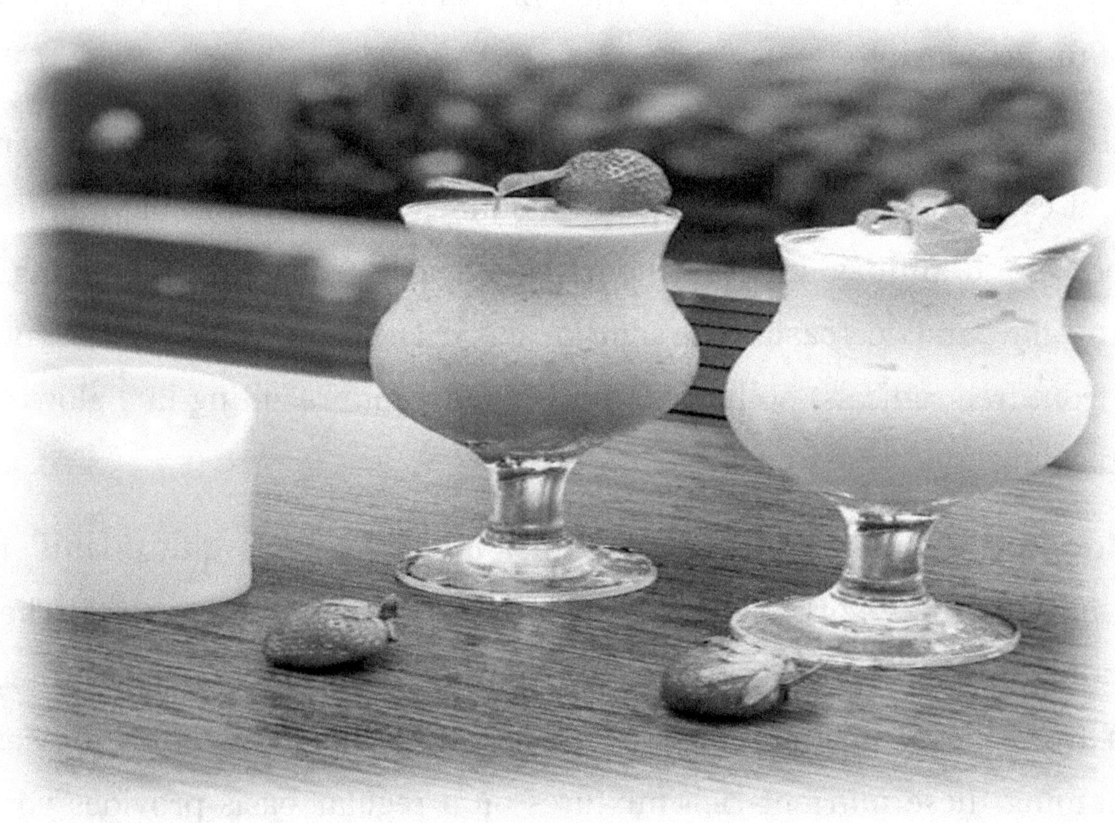

CHAPTER 2: PREPARING FOR SUCCESS

Kitchen Tools for the Perfect Smoothie

Creating tasty and nutritious alkaline smoothies does not necessitate a complex kitchen setup, but having the correct tools can help make the process easier, more efficient, and more pleasurable. Here's a look at the crucial kitchen items that will up your smoothie game:

- A high-powered blender is the heart and soul of your smoothie-making enterprise. A powerful blender, preferably with at least 1000 watts, will easily pulverize tough components such as leafy greens, frozen fruits, and fibrous vegetables, resulting in a silky-smooth texture. Choose models with several speed settings and pre-programmed smoothie functions for increased convenience.

- Measuring cups and spoons: Precision is essential when it comes to making the perfect smoothie. Measuring cups and spoons ensure that you use the proper amount of each ingredient, resulting in a balanced flavor profile and reliable results every time.

- Cutting Board and Sharp Knife: To ensure a seamless mixing experience, properly prepare your ingredients. A robust cutting board with a sharp knife will make it easy to slice fruits, vegetables, and herbs.

- Mixing Bowls: Having a few mixing bowls on hand helps you to pre-portion your components, which keeps your workstation orderly and speeds up the blending process.

- Freshly squeezed citrus juice gives many alkaline smoothies a vibrant, zesty flavor. Using a manual or electric citrus juicer, you may easily extract juice from lemons, limes, and oranges.

- Vegetable Peeler: For components such as carrots, cucumbers, and ginger, a vegetable peeler is useful for rapidly removing the outer skin.

- Mason jars or reusable cups are ideal for storing leftover smoothie ingredients or transporting your creation on the road. Look for BPA-free choices to keep your smoothies fresh and healthy.

- Straws (reusable or compostable): Drinking your smoothie using a straw can be a fun and simple way to sip on the go. Choose reusable stainless steel or glass straws, or compostable paper straws for a more environmentally friendly choice.

- Spatula: A spatula is required to extract every last drop of goodness from your blender or mixing dish.

- (Optional) Immersion Blender: If you have limited room or prefer a more compact choice, an immersion blender is a terrific alternative to a countertop blender. It allows you to blend your smoothie right in the container you intend to drink from, reducing cleanup.

With this basic kitchen equipment in your arsenal, you'll be able to make tasty, healthy, and alkalizing smoothies that will fuel your body while also pleasing your palate

Any delicious and nutritious alkaline smoothie is built on a careful selection of components. Understanding the alkalizing properties of various fruits, vegetables, and other ingredients allows you to create blends that not only satisfy your taste buds but also feed your body from the inside out.

Leafy greens:

- Kale is a nutritional powerhouse, rich in vitamins A, C, and K, as well as minerals like calcium and potassium. Its mildly bitter flavor pairs well with sweet fruits.
- Spinach: A gentler alternative to kale, spinach contains iron, magnesium, and folate. It combines easily into smoothies, creating a brilliant green color.
- Romaine lettuce, with its crisp texture and neutral flavor, adds volume and hydration to smoothies while not dominating the other components.
- Swiss chard: Swiss chard is rich in vitamins A, C, and K, as well as beta-carotene and antioxidants. Its slightly earthy flavor goes nicely with citrus fruits.

Fruits:

- Berries: Strawberries, blueberries, raspberries, and blackberries are low in sugar and strong in antioxidants, making them ideal for alkaline smoothies.
- Citrus Fruits: Lemons, limes, and grapefruits are naturally alkaline and give a refreshing zing to smoothies. Their vitamin C concentration also improves immunity.
- Tropical Fruits: Mangoes, pineapples, and papaya add sweetness and a tropical flair to your blends. They also include enzymes that help digestion.
- Apples and pear: These multipurpose fruits provide fiber and natural flavor. Choose organic variety to avoid pesticide residues.

Additional ingredients:

- Cucumber is both hydrating and cooling due to its high-water content and electrolyte concentration. It also contains silica, which promotes good skin, hair, and nails.
- Celery: This crisp vegetable is high in vitamins, minerals, and antioxidants. It also functions as a natural diuretic, aiding in the elimination of pollutants.
- Ginger is known for its anti-inflammatory effects, and it lends a spicy bite to smoothies while also soothing digestive troubles.
- Lemon or lime juice. A dash of fresh citrus juice not only brightens the flavor of your smoothie, but it also helps to keep its beautiful color.

- Fresh herbs, such as mint, basil, or cilantro, can give a distinct flavor depth to your blends.
- Spices: A bit of cinnamon, turmeric, or cayenne pepper can give your smoothie a warm and nuanced flavor.

Tips for Selecting Ingredients:

- Choose Organic: To prevent pesticides and herbicides, buy organic produce whenever feasible.
- Seasonal produce is not only fresher and tastier, but also more healthful.
- Experiment with Variety: Don't be scared to explore different ingredient combinations to find your preferred flavor profiles.
- Balance Sweetness: If your smoothie is too tart, use a natural sweetener, such as dates, honey, or maple syrup, in moderation.

Finding the correct flavor and texture balance is essential when creating a pleasant and healthful alkaline smoothie. Smoothies that nourish your health and pleasure your senses can be made by experimenting with different combinations of fresh, high-quality ingredients.

CHAPTER 3: THE 30-DAY ALKALINE SMOOTHIE DETOX PLAN

This detox plan is intended to gently transition you to an alkaline lifestyle. Every day, you'll choose a different smoothie from the categories listed, allowing you to sample a variety of flavors and health benefits. Remember to listen to your body and make adjustments as needed.

Week 1: An Introduction to Alkalinity

- Day 1: Sunrise Alkaline Booster.
- Day 2: Cucumber Mint Cleanse.
- Day 3: Avocado Lime Delight.
- Day 4: Carrot Ginger Zing.
- Day 5: Beetroot and Berry Flush.
- Day 6: Celery Pear Power.
- Day 7: Alkaline Blueberry Blast.

Week 2: Deepening the Detox

- Day 8: Kiwi Kale Kickstart.
- Day 9: Hydrate with watermelon basil. Day 10: Recharge with pineapple and spinach.
- Day 11: Berry Alkaline Fusion.
- Day 12: Tropical Alkaline Escape.
- Day 13: Green Apple Alkalinity.
- Day 14 - Sweet Spinach Revival

Week 3 - Protein and Power

- Day 15: Alkaline Antioxidant Awe.
- Days 16-18: Golden Turmeric Treat, Red Cabbage Healing Potion, and Zesty Lemon Lift.
- Day 19 - Pomegranate Cherry Chiller
- Day 20 - Flaxseed Omega Mix
- Day 21: Alkaline Nutty Adventure.

Week 4: Herbal Healing and Indulgences

- Day 22: Spirulina Protein Power.
- Day 23: Hemp Heart Harmony. Day 24: Almond Butter Bliss.
- Day 25: Chia Seed Charge.
- Days 26-28: Pumpkin Seed Elixir, Quinoa Quietude, and Sunflower Seed Sensation.

Final Days: culmination and celebration.

- Day 29: Pea Protein Perfection.
- Day 30 - Walnut Wonder

Tips for Success:

- Hydration: Drink plenty of water throughout the day to help the detoxification process.
- Mindful Eating: Pair your smoothies with a balanced, alkaline-based diet.
- Exercise: Do light to moderate exercise to improve circulation and detoxification.
- Rest: Get enough sleep to help your body's healing processes.

This detox plan will help you embrace the alkaline diet with delicious and nutritious smoothies. Adjust the plan to meet your specific health needs and preferences, and talk with a healthcare expert if you have any questions. Enjoy your journey toward alkaline health!

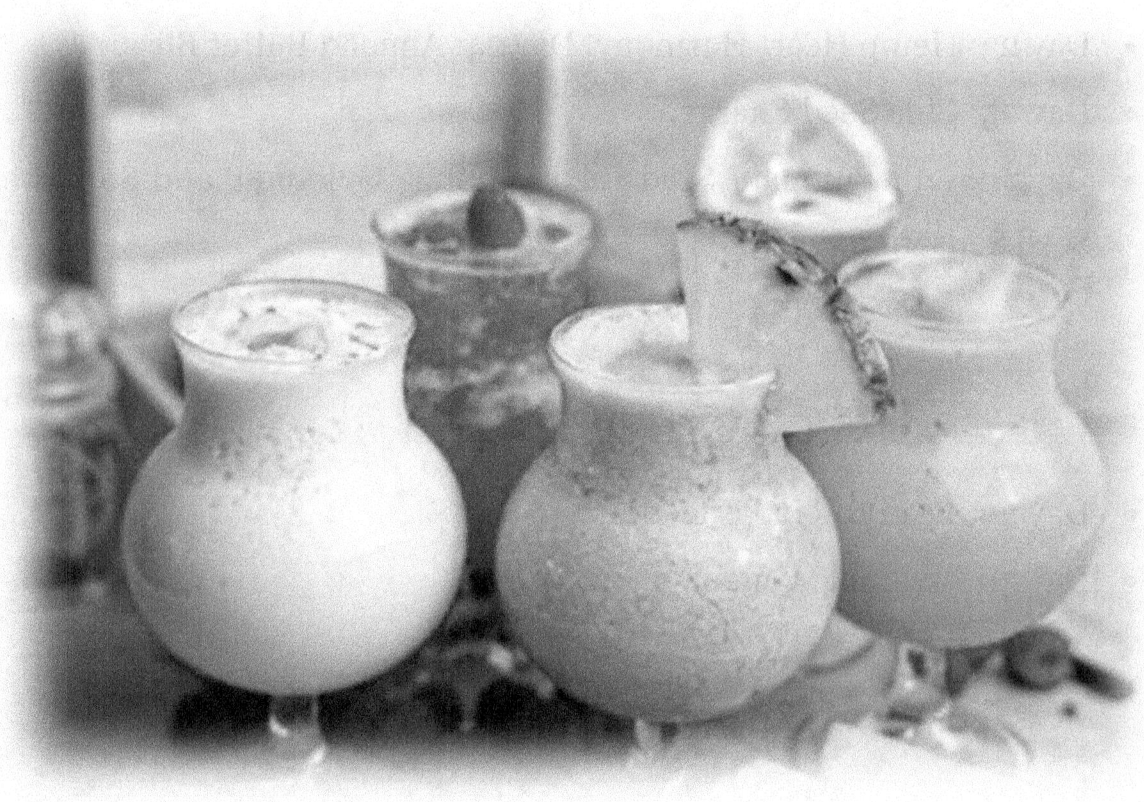

MORNING ENERGIZERS

<u>Sunrise Alkaline Booster</u>

Serves: 1

Ingredients:

• One cup of spinach.

• 1/2 cup orange juice, freshly squeezed.

• One-half banana.

• 1/4 cup carrots, chopped.

• 1/2 cup mango, cubed

• One spoonful of chia seeds.

Instructions:

• Place all items in a blender.

• Blend until smooth.

• Serve immediately.

Tip and Variations:

• To make a thicker smoothie, add frozen banana and mango.

• For an added boost, mix in a scoop of plant-based protein powder.

Nutritional Information: High in vitamin A, C, and Omega-3 fatty acids.

Cucumber-Mint Cleanse

Serves: 1

Ingredients:

• One large cucumber, peeled and sliced.

• One-half cup water

• Juice from 1 lime

• Ten mint leaves.

• One tablespoon flaxseed.

Instructions:

• Combine all ingredients in a blender.

• Blend until smooth and frothy.

• Enjoy chilled.

Tip and Variations:

• Add a sliver of ginger for a spicy kick.

• Replace flaxseed with hemp seeds for a different nutritional profile.

Nutritional Details: High in fiber and water, with cleansing qualities.

Avocado Lime Delight

Serves: 1

Ingredients:

• One ripe avocado.

• Juice from 1 lime

• One-half cup coconut water

• One-half banana.

• One tablespoon almond butter.

Instructions:

• Scoop out the avocado and add it to the blender.

• Combine the remaining ingredients.

• Blend until creamy.

Tip and Variations:

• Use a frozen banana to make a cooler smoothie.

• Top with chia seeds for extra texture and nutrition.

Nutritional Information: Packed with healthy fats, potassium, and Vitamin E.

Carrot Ginger Zing.

Serves: 1

Ingredients:

• 1 cup carrot juice, preferably freshly produced.

• One-half banana.

• 1/2-inch ginger root, peeled.

• One-quarter teaspoon turmeric powder

• One tablespoon of lemon juice.

Instructions:

• Combine all ingredients in a blender.

• Blend until smooth.

• Top with a slice of lemon.

Tip and Variations:

• For more spice, add a sprinkle of cayenne pepper.

• Add a teaspoon of raw honey if preferred.

Nutritional Information: Rich in antioxidants and Vitamin A.

Beetroot and Berry Flush.

Serves: 1

Ingredients:

• 1/2 cup beetroot, cooked and sliced

• Half cup mixed berries (strawberries, blueberries, raspberries)

• One-half banana.

• One cup of almond milk.

• One tablespoon ground flaxseed.

Instructions:

• Combine all ingredients in a blender.

• Blend until smooth.

• Serve immediately.

Tip and Variations:

• Add frozen berries for a refreshing chill.

• For more greens, mix in a handful of spinach.

Nutritional Facts: High in fiber, vitamin C, and vital minerals.

Celery Pear Power.

Serves: 1

Ingredients:

• Two stalks of celery

• One ripe pear.

• One cup of spinach.
• One tablespoon of lemon juice.

• One cup of coconut water.

Instructions:

• Chop the celery and pears into bits.

• Place all items in a blender.

• Blend until smooth.

Tip and Variations:

• Add a little slice of ginger for a spicy kick.

• For a different flavor, substitute apple instead of pear.

Nutrition Facts: A hydrating combination high in vitamins A and C.

Alkaline Blueberry Blast.

Serves: 1

Ingredients:

• 1 cup blueberries, fresh or frozen.

• One banana.

• One cup of spinach.

• One spoonful of flaxseeds

• One cup of almond milk.

Instructions:

• Combine all ingredients in a blender.

• Blend until creamy.

Tip and Variations:

• Use frozen banana to achieve a thicker consistency.

• Add a teaspoon of cinnamon for extra warmth.

Nutritional Information: Rich in antioxidants and omega-3 fatty acids.

Kiwi Kale Kickstarter

Serves: 1

Ingredients:

• Two ripe Kiwis.

• One cup of kale leaves

• One-half avocado

• One spoonful of chia seeds.

• One cup of water.

Instructions:

• Peel and slice the kiwis.

• Remove the stems from the kale.

• Combine all of the ingredients and blend until smooth.

Tip and Variations:

• For added zing, add a splash of lime juice.

• Add a drop of agave if desired.

Nutritional Facts: High in fiber and vitamin K.

Watermelon Basil Hydrator.

Serves: 1

Ingredients:

• Two cups of watermelon cubes

• 1/4 cup of fresh basil leaves.

• One tablespoon of lime juice.

• 1/2 cup of ice.

Instructions:

• Blend the watermelon, basil, and lime juice until smooth.

• Blend in ice until frosty.

Tip and Variations:

• Add a cucumber slice for extra freshness.

• To add a different herbal note, replace basil with mint.

Nutritional Information: Refreshing, high in lycopene and hydration.

Pineapple Spinach Recharge.

Serves: 1

Ingredients:

• 1 cup of pineapple pieces.

• One cup of spinach.

• One tablespoon of hemp seeds.

• One cup of coconut water.

Instructions:

• In a blender, combine pineapple, spinach, and hemp seeds.

• Add the coconut water and mix until smooth.

Tip and Variations:

• Add a few mint leaves for a refreshing twist.

• Replace pineapple for mango for a tropical twist.

Nutritional Information: An increase in vitamin C and electrolytes.

PLANT-POWERED SMOOTHIES

Berry Alkaline Fusion.

Serves: 1

Ingredients:

• 1 cup mixed berries (strawberries, raspberries, and blueberries).

• One cup of spinach.

• One tablespoon almond butter.

• One cup unsweetened almond milk.

• One teaspoon of chia seeds.

Instructions:

• Blend the berries, spinach, almond butter, and almond milk until smooth.

• Stir in the chia seeds after blending.

Tip and Variations:

• Use frozen berries to make a chilled smoothie.

• For more protein, add one scoop of plant-based protein powder.

Nutritional Information: Rich in antioxidants and vitamin C.

Tropical Alkaline Escape

Serves: 1

Ingredients:

• 1 cup of pineapple pieces.

• One banana.

• One cup of kale leaves

• One tablespoon of coconut flakes.

• One cup of coconut water.

Instructions:

• Blend the pineapple, banana, kale, and coconut water until smooth.

• Garnish with coconut flakes.

Tip and Variations:

• For a tart twist, pour in some lime juice.

• If you prefer, swap kale for spinach.

Nutritional Information: High in potassium and hydration.

Green Apple Alkalinity

Serves: 1

Ingredients:

• one green apple, cored and sliced

• 1 cup diced cucumber.

• One cup of spinach.

• One spoonful of flaxseed oil.

• One cup of cold water.

Instructions:

• In a blender, combine apples, cucumbers, spinach, and water.

• Blend until smooth, then add the flaxseed oil and mix quickly.

Tip and Variations:

• For a burst of freshness, add a handful of mint leaves.

• If preferred, sweeten with a small amount of Stevia.

Nutritional Information: Rich in fiber and healthy fats.

Sweet Spinach Revival.

Serves: 1

Ingredients:

• One cup of spinach.

• One-half avocado

• 1/2 cup mango chunks.

• One tablespoon of lemon juice.

• One cup of water.

Instructions:

• Puree spinach, avocado, mango, and water until creamy.

• Finish with a squeeze of lemon juice.

Tip and Variations:

• For a refreshing drink, add frozen mango.

• Add a teaspoon of ginger for a spicy kick.

Nutritional Information: Rich in vitamins A and E.

Alkaline Antioxidant Awe

Serves: 1

Ingredients:

• One cup mixed berry.

• One cup of spinach.

• 1/2 cup of pomegranate juice.

• One tablespoon of pumpkin seeds

• One cup of water.

Instructions:

• Blend the berries, spinach, pomegranate juice, and water until smooth.

• After blending, stir in the pumpkin seeds.

Tip and Variations:

• Add a scoop of plant-based protein to boost protein content.

• For a distinct flavor, use acai juice instead of pomegranate juice.

Nutritional Information: Rich in antioxidants and minerals.

Golden Turmeric Treat.

Serves: 1

Ingredients:

• One cup of coconut milk.

• One-half banana.

• 1/2 teaspoon of turmeric powder.

• One-quarter teaspoon cinnamon

• One spoonful of raw honey (optional).

• A pinch of black pepper.

Instructions:

• Combine all of the ingredients and blend until smooth.

• Serve immediately.

Tip and Variations:

• For more spiciness, add a teaspoon of ginger.

• To add sweetness, use dates instead of honey.

Nutritional Information: Anti-inflammatory and high in antioxidants.

Red Cabbage Healing Potion.

Serves: 1

Ingredients:

• One cup of chopped red cabbage.

• One-half cup blueberries

• One-half apple

• 1 cup water or almond milk.

• One tablespoon of lemon juice.

Instructions:

• Place all items in a blender.

• Blend until smooth.

Tip and Variations:

• Add a handful of spinach for added nutrition.

• Add stevia if desired.

Nutritional Information: Rich in vitamin C and anthocyanins.

Zesty Lemon Lift.

Serves: 1

Ingredients:

• One cup of water.

• Juice from 1 lemon

• 1/2 cucumber, sliced

• One spoonful of raw honey (optional).

• Several ice cubes.

Instructions:

• Blend water, lemon juice, cucumber, and honey until smooth.

• Add ice and mix again.

Tip and Variations:

• Add mint for a fresh twist.

• Try maple syrup as an alternate sweetener.

Nutritional Information: detoxifying and hydrating.

Pomegranate Cherry Chiller

Serves: 1

Ingredients:

• 1/2 cup pomegranate seeds.

• 1/2 cup cherries, pitted.

• One cup of coconut water.

• One tablespoon of lime juice.

• Several ice cubes.

Instructions:

• Process the pomegranate seeds, cherries, coconut water, and lime juice until smooth.

• Add ice and mix until chilled.

Tip and Variations:

• Add a scoop of plant-based protein powder for extra protein.

• If you prefer, swap the cherries with mixed berries.

Nutritional Information: High in vitamins and minerals, particularly potassium.

Flaxseed Omega Mix.

Serves: 1

Ingredients:

• One cup of spinach.

• One-half avocado

• One tablespoon of ground flaxseed

• One cup unsweetened almond milk.

• 1/2 teaspoon of vanilla extract.

Instructions:

• Combine spinach, avocado, flaxseeds, almond milk, and vanilla extract until smooth.

Tip and Variations:

• Add a banana for sweetness and thickness.

• Sprinkle with cinnamon for extra flavor.

Nutritional Information: Rich in omega-3 fatty acids and fiber.

Alkaline Nutty Adventure

Serves: 1

Ingredients:

• One cup unsweetened almond milk.

• One tablespoon almond butter.

• One-half banana.

• One spoonful of walnuts

• One-quarter teaspoon cinnamon

Instructions:

• Process almond milk, almond butter, banana, and walnuts until smooth.

• Sprinkle with cinnamon before serving.

Tip and Variations:

• Add a pinch of nutmeg for an extra spicy kick.

• Try cashew butter for a different nutty flavor.

Nutritional Info: High in healthy fats and protein.

Spirulina Protein Power

Serves: 1

Ingredients:

• One cup of coconut water.

• One banana.

• One spoonful of spirulina powder.

• One-half cup spinach

• One tablespoon of pumpkin seeds

Instructions:

• Blend the coconut water, banana, spirulina, and spinach until smooth.

• After blending, stir in the pumpkin seeds.

Tip and Variations:

• For a citrus kick, squeeze in some lemon juice.

• For added freshness, mix in a few mint leaves.

Nutritional Information: Rich in plant-based protein and iron.

Hemp Heart Harmony

Serves: 1

Ingredients:

• One cup unsweetened almond milk.

• One tablespoon of hemp hearts

• One-half avocado

• 1/2 cup mixed berries.

• 1/4 teaspoon of vanilla extract.

Instructions:

• Blend almond milk, hemp hearts, avocado, berries, and vanilla essence until smooth.

Tip and Variations:

• Use frozen berries to achieve a thicker consistency.

• If you prefer a sweeter taste, add stevia.

Nutritional Information: Rich in omega-3 fatty acids and antioxidants.

Almond Butter Bliss

Serves: 1

Ingredients:

• One cup unsweetened almond milk.

• One tablespoon almond butter.

• One ripe banana.

• 1/2 teaspoon of vanilla extract.

• One spoonful of flaxseeds

Instructions:

• Mix almond milk, almond butter, banana, and vanilla essence in a blender.

• Blend until smooth, then add the flaxseeds and blend again.

Tip and Variations:

• For a warm flavor, add a dash of cinnamon.

• Include a handful of kale for added nutrition.

Nutrition: High in fiber and monounsaturated fats.

Chia Seed Charge

Serves: 1

Ingredients:

• One cup of coconut water.

• One spoonful of chia seeds.

• 1/2 cup strawberries.

• One-half banana.

• One-quarter teaspoon lemon zest

Instructions:

• Soak the chia seeds in coconut water for ten minutes.

• Blend the soaked chia seeds, strawberries, banana, and lemon zest until smooth.

Tip and Variations:

• Add a handful of spinach for an extra serving of greens.

• Replace strawberries with blueberries for a different fruit flavor.

Nutritional Information: Rich in omega-3 fatty acids and hydration.

Pumpkin Seed Elixir

Serves: 1

Ingredients:

• One cup of spinach.

• One-quarter cup pumpkin seeds

• One-half banana.

• One cup of almond milk.

• One-quarter teaspoon cinnamon

Instructions:

• Blend spinach, pumpkin seeds, banana, and almond milk until smooth.

• Sprinkle with cinnamon before serving.

Tip and Variations:

• Soak the pumpkin seeds overnight for easy mixing.

• Add a pinch of nutmeg for a fall-themed flavor.

Nutritional Facts: High in magnesium and zinc.

Quinoa Quietude

Serves: 1

Ingredients:

• 1/4 cup cooked quinoa.

• One cup of kale leaves

• One-half avocado

• One cup of coconut water.

• One tablespoon of lemon juice.

Instructions:

• Puree the quinoa, kale, avocado, coconut water, and lemon juice until creamy.

Tip and Variations:

• Add a green apple for sweetness.

• Add chia seeds for added omega-3s.

Nutrition Facts: High in plant-based protein and fiber.

<u>Sunflower Seed Sensation.</u>

Serves: 1

Ingredients:

• One cup unsweetened almond milk.

• One-quarter cup sunflower seeds

• 1/2 ripe pear.

• One tablespoon of honey (optional)

• 1/2 teaspoon of vanilla extract.

Instructions:

• Process almond milk, sunflower seeds, pear, and vanilla essence until smooth.

• Add honey if desired.

Tip and Variations:

• For a vegan version, replace honey with maple syrup.

• Add a handful of spinach for added nutrition.

Nutritional Information: Rich in vitamin E and healthy fats.

Pea Protein Perfection

Serves: 1

Ingredients:

• One cup of coconut water.

• One scoop of pea protein powder.

• One-half banana.

• 1/4 cup of cucumber slices.

• One tablespoon of mint leaves.

Instructions:

• Mix the coconut water, pea protein powder, banana, cucumber, and mint until smooth.

Tip and Variations:

• To make a cooler smoothie, freeze the banana ahead.

• For a refreshing twist, pour in some lime juice.

Nutritional Information: A great source of plant-based protein and water.

Walnut Wonder

Serves: 1

Ingredients:

• One cup unsweetened almond milk.

• One-quarter cup walnuts

• Half an apple, cored and sliced

• One-half teaspoon cinnamon

• One tablespoon ground flaxseed.

Instructions:

• Blend almond milk, walnuts, apple, and cinnamon until smooth.

• Stir in the ground flaxseed after blending.

Tip and Variations:

• Soak walnuts overnight for a smoother mix.

• Add a pinch of clove for a spicy kick.

Nutritional Information: Rich in omega-3 fatty acids and antioxidants.

HEALING HERBAL SMOOTHIES

Minty Alkaline Refresher

Serves: 1

Ingredients:

• One cup of spinach.

• One-half cucumber

• Ten fresh mint leaves.

• Juice from 1 lime

• One cup of water.

Instructions:

• Process the spinach, cucumber, mint leaves, lime juice, and water until smooth.

Tip and Variations:

• Add a couple pieces of ginger for a spicy kick.

• Add a drizzle of agave nectar if preferred.

Nutritional Information: Refreshing, high in Vitamin K, and hydrating.

Herbal Antioxidant Blast.

Serves: 1

Ingredients:

• 1/2 cup mixed berries.

• 1/4 cup of fresh parsley.

• One tablespoon of lemon juice.

• 1 cup green tea, chilled

Instructions:

• Blend the berries, parsley, lemon juice, and green tea until smooth.

Tip and Variations:

• For added taste, brew the green tea with a bag of herbal tea.

• Use frozen berries to make a chilled smoothie.

Nutritional Information: Rich in antioxidants and flavonoids.

Basil Berry Medley

Serves: 1

Ingredients:

• One cup strawberry.

• One-half banana.

• 1/4 cup of fresh basil leaves.

• One cup of almond milk.

Instructions:

• Combine strawberries, banana, basil leaves, and almond milk until smooth.

Tip and Variations:

• For a lighter version, use coconut water instead of almond milk.

• For added fiber, add 1 tablespoon chia seeds.

Nutritional Information: High in Vitamin C and Manganese.

Thyme & Plum Potion

Serves: 1

Ingredients:

• Two ripe plums, pitted

• 1/2 cup of red grapes.

• One teaspoon of fresh thyme leaves.

• One cup of water.

Instructions:

• Puree the plums, grapes, thyme leaves, and water until smooth.

Tip and Variations:

• For more tartness, add a splash of lemon juice.

• Add a teaspoon of raw honey if necessary.

Nutritional Information: Rich in Vitamin A and dietary fiber.

Rosemary Citrus Surprise

Serves: 1

Ingredients:

• One orange, peeled and seeded

• 1/2 grapefruit, peeled and seeded.

• One teaspoon of fresh rosemary.

• One cup of water.

Instructions:

• Blend the orange, grapefruit, rosemary, and water until smooth.

Tip and Variations:

• For a sweeter flavor, add a tiny apple.

• To achieve a frosty texture, freeze the citrus fruits ahead.

Nutritional Information: Rich in Vitamin C and bioflavonoids.

Lavender Blueberry Calm.

Serves: 1

Ingredients:

• One cup blueberry.

• One teaspoon of dried lavender flowers.

• One cup of almond milk.

• One-half banana.

Instructions:

• Blend the blueberries, lavender, almond milk, and banana until smooth.

Tip and Variations:

• For a sweeter smoothie, add a small amount of raw honey.

• To make a chilled version, use frozen blueberries.

Nutritional Information: High in antioxidants and recognized for its relaxing effects.

Sage Strawberry Serenity.

Serves: 1

Ingredients:

• One cup strawberry.

• One-half banana.

• One teaspoon of fresh sage leaves.

• One cup of coconut water.

Instructions:

• Blend the strawberries, banana, sage leaves, and coconut water until smooth.

Tip and Variations:

• Add a handful of spinach for added nutrition.

• Replace sage with basil for a different herbal flavor.

Nutritional Facts: High in vitamin C and potassium.

Chamomile-Peach Comfort

Serves: 1

Ingredients:

• Two ripe, pitted peaches

• 1 cup of brewed chamomile tea, cooled

• 1/2 teaspoon of vanilla extract.

• One tablespoon ground flaxseed.

Instructions:

• Combine peaches, chamomile tea, vanilla extract, and milled flaxseed until smooth.

Tip and Variations:

• If you prefer a sweeter taste, add stevia.

• Add a pinch of cinnamon for a toasty flavoring.

Nutritional Information: Soothes and aids digestion.

Lemon Balm Bliss

Serves: 1

Ingredients:

• One cup of spinach.

• One-half cucumber

• One tablespoon of lemon balm leaves.

• Juice from 1 lemon

• One cup of water.

Instructions:

• Process spinach, cucumber, lemon balm, lemon juice, and water until smooth.

Tip and Variations:

• Add a sliver of ginger for a spicy kick.

• For a different, more refreshing flavor, replace lemon balm with mint.

Nutritional Information: Refreshing and stress-reducing.

Parsley Pear Purify

Serves: 1

Ingredients:

• One ripe pear.

• 1/4 cup of parsley leaves.

• One cup of kale leaves

• One tablespoon of lemon juice.

• One cup of water.

Instructions:

• Process the pear, parsley, kale, lemon juice, and water until smooth.

Tip and Variations:

• Add a green apple for extra sweetness.

• To add electrolytes, use coconut water instead of ordinary water.

Nutritional Information: Detoxifying, high in vitamins A and C.

Chocolate Alkaline Indulgence.

Serves: 1

Ingredients:

• One cup of almond milk.

• One tablespoon of raw cacao powder.

• One-half avocado

• One tablespoon of pure maple syrup.

• 1/2 teaspoon of vanilla extract.

Instructions:

• Process almond milk, cacao powder, avocado, maple syrup, and vanilla extract until smooth.

Tip and Variations:

• Enhance the chocolate flavor with a pinch of sea salt.

• For more protein, add a scoop of almond protein powder.

Nutritional Value: High in healthy fats and magnesium.

Sweet Alkaline Dream.

Serves: 1

Ingredients:

• One cup of coconut water.

• One-half banana.

• 1/2 cup mango chunks.

• One tablespoon of coconut flakes.

• One-half teaspoon cinnamon

Instructions:

• Blend the coconut water, banana, mango, and cinnamon until smooth.

• Garnish with coconut flakes.

Tip and Variations:

• Add frozen fruit to make the smoothie cooler and thicker.

• To add spice, sprinkle with nutmeg.

Nutritional Information: Rich in vitamins A and C.

Vanilla Bean Velvet

Serves: 1

Ingredients:

• One cup unsweetened almond milk.

• One-half scraped vanilla bean

• One-half banana.

• One tablespoon of hemp seeds.

• 1/2 teaspoon of almond extract.

Instructions:

• Combine almond milk, vanilla bean, banana, and almond extract until smooth.

• Add hemp seeds after blending.

Tip and Variations:

• Add a date for natural sweetness.

• Replace hemp seeds with chia seeds for a different texture.

Nutritional Information: Rich in plant-based protein and omega-3 fatty acids.

Cacao Coconut Concoction

Serves: 1

Ingredients:

• One cup of coconut milk.

• One tablespoon of cacao nibs.

• One-half banana.

• One tablespoon of shredded coconut.

• 1/2 teaspoon of cacao powder.

Instructions:

• Process the coconut milk, cacao nibs, banana, and cacao powder until smooth.

• Top with shredded coconut.

Tip and Variations:

• To achieve a frosty texture, freeze the banana first.

• Add a teaspoon of almond butter for extra richness.

Nutritional Information: Rich in antioxidants and good fats.

Maple Cinnamon Marvel

Serves: 1

Ingredients:

• One cup oat milk.

• One tablespoon of pure maple syrup.

• One-half teaspoon cinnamon

• Half an apple, cored and cut

• One spoonful of flaxseeds

Instructions:

• Blend oat milk, maple syrup, cinnamon, apple, and flaxseeds until smooth.

Tip and Variations:

• Add a pinch of ground ginger for a warming effect.

• For a distinct flavor profile, substitute pears for apples.

Nutritional Information: High fiber content and heart-healthy omega-3s.

Alkaline Apple Pie

Serves: 1

Ingredients:

• One apple, cored and sliced

• One cup unsweetened almond milk.

• One-half teaspoon cinnamon

• 1/4 teaspoon nutmeg.

• One spoonful of soaked almonds.

Instructions:

• Combine all of the ingredients and blend until smooth.

Tip and Variations:

• Add a date for natural sweetness.

• Add a sprinkle of ground flaxseed for added fiber.

Nutritional Facts: High in fiber and warming spices.

Berry Cheesecake Charm.

Serves: 1

Ingredients:

• One cup mixed berry.

• 1/2 cup cashews (soaked for 2 hours)

• One cup unsweetened almond milk.

• 1/2 teaspoon of vanilla extract.

Instructions:

• Combine the berries, soaked cashews, almond milk, and vanilla essence until smooth.

Tip and Variations:

• Use frozen berries to make a thicker smoothie.

• Sprinkle with a few whole berries on top.

Nutritional Information: Rich in antioxidants and good fats.

Peach Cobbler Paradise

Serves: 1

Ingredients:

• Two ripe peaches, pitted and sliced

• One cup unsweetened almond milk.

• One-half teaspoon cinnamon

• One spoonful rolled oats.

Instructions:

• Blend peaches, almond milk, cinnamon, and oats until smooth.

Tip and Variations:

• Add a pinch of ginger for a spicy kick.

• If you like a sweeter taste, sweeten with stevia.

Nutritional Information: High in vitamin C and fiber.

Banana Nut Bread Bliss.

Serves: 1

Ingredients:

• One banana.

• One cup unsweetened almond milk.

• One-quarter teaspoon cinnamon

• One spoonful of walnuts

• 1/4 teaspoon of vanilla extract.

Instructions:

• Blend banana, almond milk, cinnamon, walnuts, and vanilla extract until smooth.

Tip and Variations:

• Use a frozen banana for a creamier, colder texture.

• Add chia seeds for additional nutrition.

Nutrition: High in potassium and omega-3s.

Carob Cherry Cream.

Serves: 1

Ingredients:

• 1 cup pitted cherries.

• One cup unsweetened almond milk.

• One tablespoon of carob powder.

• One-half banana.

Instructions:

• Blend the cherries, almond milk, carob powder, and banana until smooth.

Tip and Variations:

• For added protein, add a spoonful of hemp seeds.

• To make a frosty treat, freeze the cherries ahead.

Nutritional Information: High fiber content and naturally sweet.

Tips for Long-Term Alkaline Health

Starting an alkaline diet is more than just a quick remedy; it's a lifestyle shift that can have a significant impact on your overall health and well-being. To get the benefits of this nourishing style of eating, develop long-term habits that support your alkaline balance and general vigor.

Here are some important strategies for preserving long-term alkaline health.

Embrace the 80/20 rule:

- Aim for an 80% alkaline, 20% acidic diet. This provides versatility and enjoyment while keeping a primarily alkaline atmosphere.
- Don't worry about occasional indulgences. Enjoy a slice of pizza or a piece of chocolate cake on occasion without feeling guilty! The key is moderation and balance.

Focus on Variety:

- Don't limit yourself to just a few components. To provide a diverse spectrum of nutrients, eat a variety of alkaline fruits, vegetables, nuts, seeds, and legumes.
- Be inventive with your recipes. Experiment with various Flavors, textures, and combinations to make your alkaline journey interesting and delightful.

Plan ahead:

- Preparing meals on weekends or evenings ensures that you have healthy, alkaline options available all week.
- Alkaline basics such as leafy greens, fruits, vegetables, nuts, seeds, and healthy fats should be kept on hand in the fridge and pantry.
- Pack alkaline snacks for on-the-go nutrition.

Stay hydrated:

- Make water the major beverage. Aim for 8-10 glasses of filtered water per day to aid with detoxification, hydration, and alkaline balance.
- To enhance flavor and benefits, infuse your water with alkaline-boosting foods such as lemon, cucumber, or mint.

Listen to your body.

- Consider how different foods and activities affect your mood. If something doesn't sit well with you, don't force it.
- Adjust your routine as needed. Your body's needs may shift over time, so be adaptable and modify your alkaline routines accordingly.

Seek Support:

- Join a community of like-minded people who share your enthusiasm for alkaline living. This can bring motivation, inspiration, and useful information.
- Consider working with a holistic nutritionist or health coach who can provide tailored advice and support along your journey.

Make it a lifestyle.

- Don't think of alkaline living as a rigorous diet or a transitory solution. Accept it as a way of life that benefits your health, mind, and spirit.
- Celebrate your accomplishments and enjoy the trip!

By adopting these recommendations into your daily routine, you can develop a long-term alkaline lifestyle that promotes health, vitality, and well-being.

Remember that the journey to alkaline health is a marathon, not a sprint. Be patient, gentle to yourself, and enjoy the process of nurturing your body from the inside out.

<u>FAQs</u>

Q: What is an alkaline diet?

A: The alkaline diet emphasizes eating foods that are thought to promote an alkaline environment in your body. This contains plenty of fruits, vegetables, nuts, seeds, and legumes, as well as reducing acidic items such as processed meals, sugar, red meat, and milk.

Q: What are the benefits of consuming alkaline smoothies?

A: Alkaline smoothies have various benefits, including:

- Balancing your body's pH
- Increasing energy levels
- Aiding digestion.
- Promoting detoxification.
- Supporting weight management
- Providing necessary nourishment.

Q. Are all fruits and veggies alkaline?

A: While most fruits and vegetables are alkaline-forming, some, such as citrus fruits, are acidic in nature but have an alkalizing effect on the body when processed.

Q: Can I have alkaline smoothies every day?

A: Absolutely! Including alkaline smoothies in your daily routine is an excellent approach to fuel your body and promote overall wellness.

Q: Can alkaline smoothies help you lose weight?

A: While alkaline smoothies are not a miracle weight reduction cure, they can help you achieve your objectives by supplying important nutrients, increasing fullness, and decreasing cravings for unhealthy snacking.

Q: Are there any side effects from drinking alkaline smoothies?

A: The majority of people can safely consume alkaline smoothies. However, if you have any underlying health conditions, you should always check your doctor before making significant dietary changes.

Q: Can I mix protein powder into my alkaline smoothie?

A: Yes! Adding plant-based protein powder, such as hemp, pea, or rice protein, will boost the nutritional value of your smoothie and keep you feeling filled longer.

Q: How do I make my alkaline smoothies more flavorful?

A: Try different combinations of fruits, veggies, herbs, and spices. A squeeze of lemon or lime juice can brighten the dish, while a dash of ginger or cinnamon will add warmth and depth.

Q: Can I freeze alkaline smoothies?

A: Yes, you may freeze any leftover smoothie in a freezer-safe container for a quick and easy snack later. Just make sure there's enough space at the top for the smoothie to expand as it freezes.

Q: Is it better to juice or blend alkaline smoothies?

A: Blending is favoured for alkaline smoothies because it preserves the fiber found in fruits and vegetables, which is essential for digestion and blood sugar regulation.

I hope these FAQs have solved some of your questions regarding alkaline smoothies. The route to alkaline health is unique to each individual, so listen to your body, try different recipes, and see what works best for you.

CONCLUSION

Congratulations! You've completed this alkaline smoothie experience, and I hope you feel inspired, energized, and ready to go on a road to a healthier, more vibrant you.

As you've discovered, alkaline smoothies are more than simply a tasty beverage; they're also an effective tool for improving your health from the inside out. You may achieve your greatest potential and live a life full of energy, vitality, and joy by fueling your body with nutrient-dense foods, restoring balance, and adopting a holistic approach to health.

Remember that the journey to alkaline health is personal. Enjoy the freedom to personalize your lifestyle to your specific requirements and tastes. Experiment with recipes, listen to your body's cues, and don't be hesitant to try something new. The opportunities are limitless, and the benefits are truly life-changing.

As you continue on your alkaline smoothie journey, I encourage you to share your achievements and challenges with others. Spread the word about the benefits of alkaline living, and encourage those around you to adopt a healthy lifestyle.

If this book has benefited you in any way, I would be grateful if you could post a favourable review and provide honest feedback. Your remarks not only mean a lot to me, but they also help others understand the transformative potential of alkaline smoothies.

Thank you for joining me on my path toward better health. May your blender be always full, your smoothies bursting with taste, and your life filled with radiant well-being.